BOOST YOUR HEALTH LIFE

WITH

GINSENG

ROOTS & HERBS

GUIDE

DR. ALICE ONOFUA

TABLE OF CONTENTS

Introduction

And God said, *"..Behold I have given you every herb bearing seed which is upon the face of all the earth, and every tree in which is the fruit of a tree yielding seed; to you it shall become meat."* Gen. 1:30.

It could then be deduced from the aforesaid that God desire a healthy life for son of men. One of the gifts of nature to mankind to enhance their well-being is Ginseng. Its original name is "man-root" because the root resembles the shape of human body. It is an herbal supplements that has been in use for centuries in Chinese medicine.

Ginseng is commonly touted for its antioxidant and anti-inflammatory effects. It could also help regulate blood sugar level and have benefits for some cancer and diabetic patients.

Furthermore, it has the potential to strengthen immune system, enhance brain function, fight fatigue, and improve symptoms of erectile dysfunction (ED) and several others you will find in the course of reading this book.

Ginseng can be consumed raw, steamed, made as a tea or be added as spice to diet through its extracts, capsules or powder form.

Give your health a boost!

HISTORY OF GINSENG

According to the American Botanical Council, the use of herbal supplements in the US has been steadily increasing. Sales of these products in 2017 totaled more than $8 billion. As these products become more popular, we should ask ourselves: are they actually safe and effective?

Ginseng, a regularly top-selling herbal supplement, comes from the root part of several plant species in the *Panax* genus. The most common type of Ginseng supplement comes from *Panax ginseng*, which roughly translates to "all-healing man-root." It is also called Asian Ginseng, Chinese Ginseng, or Korean Ginseng. Other sources of ginseng include American Ginseng (*Panax quinquefolius*) and Tianqi Ginseng (*Panax notoginseng*). This root has been used for thousands of years as part of traditional Chinese medicine and is said to improve physical and mental performance and increase the body's ability to respond to stress.

Outside of the Ginseng supplements available for purchase over-the-counter, Ginseng can be consumed in many different forms. The raw root can be peeled and chewed, soaked in wine to make an extract for drinking, or boiled to make a tea. Dried Ginseng can be soaked or boiled until it is soft and then stewed to make an extract for drinking. Ginseng is a common ingredient in many energy drinks and teas and it is a regular addition to Asian cuisine.

The desire to use natural products that are not mass-produced is understandable. However, it is important to acknowledge that these herbal and homemade treatments come with their own risks. No two Ginseng roots are the same, and there is no way to guarantee how much (if any) active ingredient from the Ginseng is being ingested when using the natural root.

In general, Ginseng use is well tolerated, but some patients experience side effects when taking it. Side effects associated with both Asian and American Ginseng include nervousness, insomnia, changes in blood pressure, breast pain, vaginal bleeding, vomiting, diarrhea, and mania. There have been rare reports of patients experiencing severe symptoms like inflammation of the arteries in the brain (cerebral arteritis), severe skin reactions (Stevens-Johnson syndrome), inflammation of the liver (cholestatic hepatitis), and anaphylactic allergic reactions.

Ginseng has also been shown to interact with other herbal products, prescribed medications, and foods. This list includes caffeine, alcohol, blood-thinners, and medications for the treatment of HIV, diabetic medications, immunosuppressants, antidepressants, bitter orange, ephedra, and bitter mallow. Avoiding these interactions is why it is important to speak to your physician and Pharmacist before taking products like Ginseng.

There are a few studies showing that Ginseng use is possibly effective in improving cognitive function and Alzheimer's disease, chronic obstructive pulmonary disease, influenza, fatigue related to multiple sclerosis, erectile dysfunction, premature ejaculation, and sexual arousal. This research is preliminary or limited in many of these studies and further study is needed.

In 2015, the New York Attorney General's office tested herbal products from four major retailers (GNC, Target, Walmart, and Walgreens). Ginseng supplements from each of these retailers were included in the testing. They found that 79% of the herbal products tested did not contain any of the plants listed on the ingredient labels and many contained unlisted contaminants from other plants. You can check alerts provided by the Food and Drug Administration to ensure that there are no active warnings or recalls on the product you are interested in using.

Chapter One

WHAT IS GINSENG?

Ginseng refers to eleven different varieties of a short, slow-growing plant with flesh root: Slow-growing in the sense that it takes between 3-5years to grow.

The root resembles the shape of human body and that's where it derived the original name - "man-root." Ancient Chinese doctrines state ***"that a plant that resembles a human body part will definitely have a healing effect on that body part."*** Therefore, it is believed that Ginseng is able to restore harmony to the whole body and also enhance wellbeing.

Ginseng is one of the most popular herbal remedies. The herb consists of a light-coloured, forked shaped root, a relatively long stalk and green leaves with an oval shape and bright red berries. However, it is only the root that has medicinal value.

Ginseng contains complex carbohydrates called ***"saponins"*** for it possesses anti-inflammatory antioxidant and anti-cancer elements.

Ginseng is sometimes called ***"adaptogen"*** for it normalizes bodily function depending on individual's needs. However, taking too much "adaptogen" has side effects from headache to digestive issues – sleep, high blood pressure, dizziness, heart palpitations and more.

TYPES OF GINSENG

There are different species of Ginseng. They vary in their concentrations of active Compound and effect on the body:

AMERICAN AND CANADIAN GINSENG. Known as *Panax quinquefolius*

ASIAN OR KOREAN RED GINSENG. Known as *Panas Ginseng*

Canadian Ginseng is the most balanced of all the Ginseng varieties and it is known to have twice the concentration of *ginsenosides* of Korean Ginseng.

Furthermore, Canadian Ginseng is considered to be more relaxing and known to increase the "ying" energy and has a cooling effect on the body.

Korean Ginseng is the Asian root which has a warming effect on the body. However, it is not recommended for menopausal women or people with high blood pressure or hypertension.

It is known to increase the "yang" energy and is considered most suitable for males and older people because of the invigorating effect.

COMPOUNDS/COMPONENTS OF GINSENG

Ginseng contains two significant compounds – *ginsenosides* and *gintonin.* They complement one another to provide health benefits.

Ginseng contains a number of active ingredients called ginsenosides as well as sugars, amino acids, vitamins and minerals.

The gensenosides are the most active ingredient and 25 different types have been found. Only 6 of them are thought to have any therapeutic significance. Research suggests that the ginsenosides that may appear inactive actually help to make the "active" ginsenosides more soluble, more easily absorb-able and more bio-available to the body.

CLASSIFICATIONS OF GINSENG

Ginseng can be classified into three ways. This depends on how long it is grown.

- FRESH - This is harvested before 4 years.
- WHITE - This is harvested between 4 – 6 years.
- RED   - This is harvested after 6 years.

Chapter Two

HEALTH BENEFITS OF GINSENG

Ginseng is reputed to have multiple health benefits as we shall later find out in this book.

Ginseng has traditionally been taken to aid wide range of medical conditions.

Both American Ginseng and Asian Ginseng are believed to provide the following health benefits.

1. REDUCES STRESS

The phenomenon of stress is often cited as the reason for various diseases.

Changes in the autonomic nervous system and in the hormonal balance which occur during the stress reaction can at high intensity and long duration – certainly cause physical damage. This is proven for example for the development of cardiovascular diseases.

With the help of the Ginseng root, the body is able to react faster to the different stress triggers and to deal with them in a better way. The increased resistance delays exhaustion and stress related diseases and possibly even prevent them.

Ginseng causes less stress hormones to be formed and existing ones to be metabolized faster.

2. HELPS THE BRAIN

Ginseng stimulates the brain with the help of an *"electroensephalogram"* (EEG). One can measure which cells work and how intensively they do that. Biochemical laboratory studies show that the cells have an increased activity with increasing Ginseng dose.

3. FIGHTS FATIQUE

It is interesting to note that Ginseng may help fight fatigue and enhance physical activity by lowering oxidative damage and increasing energy production in cells.

4. LOWERS BLOOD PRESSURE

Ginseng seems to be beneficial in the control of blood glucose in people either with or without diabetics.
American and Asian Ginseng have been shown to improve pancreatic cell function, boost insulin production and enhance the uptake of blood sugar in tissues.

Fermented red Ginseng may help increase insulin production, enhance blood sugar uptake on cells and provide antioxidant protection.

5. IMPROVES PERFORMANCE OF ATHLETES.

Ginseng improves performance under stress.

The performance of Athletes increases with the intake. It optimize the metabolic process, this active people can make better use of their energy.

Specifically, improved muscle oxygen uptake and uthization, increases heart bear volume and a decrease of lactose concentration in the blood were observed.

In essence, with Ginseng, there is no reason for doping to boost physical performance.

6. IMPROVES ERECTILE DYSFUNCTION

Research has shown that Ginseng may be a useful alternative for the treatment of erectile dysfunction in men (ED).

It seems that compound in it may protect against oxidative stress in blood vessels and tissues in the penis and help restore normal function.

Furthermore, studies have proved that Ginseng may promote the production **nitric oxide** – a compound that improves muscle relaxation in the penis and increases blood circulation.

Ginseng may improve symptoms of erectile dysfunctions by decreasing oxidative stress in tissues and enhancing blood flow in penile muscles.

7. HELPS CANCER PATIENTS

Studies show that Ginseng may strengthen the immune system in cancer patients, and even enhance the effects of certain vaccinations.

Ginseng is helpful in reducing the risk of certain cancer.

Ginsenosides have been shown to help reduce inflammation and provide antioxidant protection.
The cell cycle is the process by which cells normally grow and divide. Ginsenosides could benefit this cycle by preventing abnormal cell production and growth.

A review of several studies concluded that people who take Ginseng may have a 16% lower risk of developing cancer.

Moreover, an observational study suggested that people taking Ginseng could less likely to developing certain types of cancer such as lip, mouth , esophagus, stomach, colon, liver and lung cancer than those who do not take it.

Ginseng may also improve the health of patients undergoing chemotherapy, reduce side effects and enhance the effect of some treatment drugs.

Similarly, Ginsenosides in Ginseng seem to regulate inflammation, provide antioxidant protection and maintain the health of cells, which could help decrease the risk of certain kinds of cancer. Nevertheless, more research is needed.

8. PREVENTS/ALLEVIATES SIDE EFFECT OF CANCER

Research has linked positive association of Ginseng used in breast cancer survivors.

Findings show that patients who used Ginseng prior to cancer treatment had a higher rate of survival, with use after treatment increasing quality of life.

Other studies have found that the fatigue associated with cancer treatment was lessened through the use of Ginseng.

9. TREATS DIABETES.

Studies show that Ginseng extracts help by providing antioxidant protection that reduces free radicals in the cells of those with diabetes.

10. GENERAL HEALTH BENEFITS TO WOMEN

Many women take Ginseng during the menopausal years to reduce hot flashes, headaches, insomnia, irritability and other discomforts.

Ginseng is well equipped to balance, tone, and support the hormone system during this time of change.

11. POTENTIAL NATURAL STIMULANT FOR FOCUS AND ATTENTION

Ginseng act as a natural stimulant and is prized for its effect for focus and attention. It is touted as the earlier pharmacological treatment for ADHD.

One study, however, discovered that Ginseng did have positive effect on children with ADHD and another Study found that it also has a positive impact on Alzheimer's.

Chapter Three

FAST FACTS ON GINSENG

Ginsenosides is a chemical component found in Ginseng, it is claimed that the component is responsible for the chemical effects of the herbs.

Ginseng products can vary in their quality and medicinal properties, therefore, as said ealier, there are different types and some products contain a small or negligible amount of Ginseng and some contain other substance not found in others. It thus makes it necessary to check the ingredients before buying.

Ginseng has beneficial antioxidant anti – inflammatory effects.

Some test tubes studies have shown that Ginseng extracts and ginsenosides compounds could inhibit inflammation and increase antioxidant capacity in cells.

Another test tube found that Korean red Ginseng extract reduces inflammation and improves antioxidant activity in skin cells from people with eczema.

Ginseng is meant to be used as a supplement: An occasional additive not part of dietary routine.

Ginseng has no natural food sources, it is ometimes added to energy drinks and foods.

HOW TO USE GINSENG

Ginseng root can be consumed in many ways:

It can be eaten raw or can be lightly steamed to soften it. It can also be stewed in water to make tea. To do this, just add hot water to freshly sliced Ginseng and allow it steep for several minutes.

It can also be soaked in wine to make an extract for drinking.

It can be added to various recipes like soup and stir –fry's too.

The extract can be found in powder, tablet, capsule and oil forms.

Study showed that the pharmacological effect is far more potent when used as a tea, tincture or powder than when infused, fried or eaten raw.

The dosage to be taken depends on the condition the user wants to use it for; however, it is advisable to consult a Doctor.

Ginseng extracts that contains 2-3% total ginsenosides is better taken before meals to increase absorption and optimal benefits and results.

Chapter Four

SIDE EFFECTS

Natural does not always mean 'safe'.
Like all medicines, herbal products and supplements are expected to have some side effects and Ginseng is no exception. Some side effects are related to the natural toxicity of the plants they come from or the manufacturers.

Ginseng is well tolerated but some patients experience side effects when taking it. That is to say the following notable side effects may occur when not taking according to prescription or medical advice.

- Headache
- Sleep problem
- Digestive problem
- Charges to blood pressure and blood sugar
- Irritability
- Nervousness
- Blurred vision
- A serve skin reaction
- Eczema
- Diarrhea
- Bleeding
- Dizziness

- Dry mouth
- A decreased heart rate
- Convulsion and seizures
- Delirium
- Women may also experience swollen breasts and vaginal bleeding.

PRECAUTIONS

According to research, Ginseng appears to be safe and should not produce any serious adverse effects. However, people taking certain medications should pay attention to possible drug interactions.

In this view, it is advisable that diabetic patients should monitor their blood sugar level closely when using Ginseng to ensure these levels do not go too low. Furthermore, Ginseng may reduce the effectiveness of anticoagulant drugs.

Due to lack of safety studies, Ginseng is not recommended for children, pregnant or those who plan to become pregnant soon or those breast feeding.

Ginseng should be taken in the professional advice of a Doctor because there is evidence suggesting that the extended use of Ginseng could decrease its effectiveness in the body.

It is therefore advised that users should follow instructions and do not take more than the recommended dose.

Similarly users should consult the Doctor before using any natural product. Some products may not mix well with drugs or other natural products.

Furthermore, it is advised that users should not use Ginseng when having health problem that are sensitive to known hormones. For example: breast cancer, prostate cancer or endometriosis.

INTERACTIONS
Medical Doctors have advised against mixing Ginseng with a class of antidepressants called Monoamine oxidaze inhibitors (MAOLs).

They said taking the two together can cause maniac episodes and tremors.

Ginseng can alter the effects of Blood pressure, diabetes and heart medications including calcium channel blockers such as nifedipin.
Therefore, it is not advisable to mix Ginseng and heart medications without first consulting a Doctor.

The herb can also increase the risk of bleeding when taken with blood thinners such as warfarin or aspirin.

Ginseng may intensify the effects of caffeine and other stimulants, thereby leading to a rapid heartbeat and possible sweating or insomnia. It could also possibly cancel out the pain-killing effects of morphine.

Frequently asked questions on Ginseng

The main active ingredients of Ginseng root are called ginsenosides. They belong to the substance group of saponins. They are identified by abbreviations, each beginning with an R. In the 1980s, 13 ginsenosides were known, and by now almost 40 ginsenosides are described in the literature.

That the "man-like root" both revive and calm can be traced back to the interplay of the various ginsenosides. For example, the two best-studied ginsenosides, Rg1 and Rb1, are known to be "antagonists" that harmoniously complement each other, as well as Ying and Yang in Chinese medicine: Rg1 raises blood pressure, has a stimulating effect and enhances performance and responsiveness, Rb1 lowers blood pressure, soothes excitement and helps to relax.

In addition to the ginsenosides, numerous vitamins and minerals are contained in the Ginseng root, each contributing to the health-promoting effect.

The complex effect of Ginseng on the human body ultimately results from the complex composition of the active ingredients in the root. As usually it also applies here: The lot is more than the sum of its parts!

For whom is Ginseng recommended?

Ginseng can in principle be taken by anyone and regardless of age. It is recommended especially for the prevention of typical "common diseases", such as diabetes, cardiovascular diseases or cancer, for prevention of the symptoms of old age and in the recovery phase after a serious illness. The healthier and well-toned your body, the more balanced your soul and psyche, the less you perceive the effect. But Ginseng works in secrecy: A healthy body does not seem to respond to Ginseng, but it can handle it much better when it comes to stresses and strains than it would without Ginseng. A regular Ginseng cure is especially recommended for:

- Stressed people (Manager, working mothers, Teachers, et.al.)
- Shifters (Nurses, Policemen, et.al.)
- Seniors
- Athletics
- Patients in recovery after surgery
- People who are going through a difficult phase. People who want to prevent stress-related widespread diseases.

When do I feel the effect?

In contrast to synthetic drugs, which usually have a very targeted and rapid effect, the Ginseng needs some time to make the body feel its regulating effect. But the effect then lasts for a long time extending the intake period, so that you usually get by with one to two Ginseng cures a year. The healthier and more balanced you are, the less you feel an immediate effect. However, if your metabolism or your inner life is out of balance, you will recognize a noticeable effect about two to three weeks after starting the Ginseng treatment.

How do I take Ginseng best?

Generally, a 100-day-cure is recommended with a daily dose of one to two grams of ginseng root with a minimum ginsenoside content of 0.4 percent (Ph.Eur.). If you use Ginseng SL from FloraFarm, one gram of Ginseng root (equivalent to two capsules of ginseng SL, each containing 167 mg of ginseng extract) per day is usually sufficient, as our Ginseng has been shown to contain more than twice the prescribed minimum content of ginsenosides.

Taking Ginseng as capsule:

Take two capsules in the morning, then you are ready for the day!

Taking Ginseng as root:

If you like the original and the bittersweet taste of the root, we recommend one gram of the dried root in the first half of the day: Before swallowing, allow the root parts to melt in the mouth for as long as possible until they are completely soft. Thus, the active ingredients are optimally absorbed through the oral mucosa.

Whether root or capsule, the effect is the same! The active ingredients are either absorbed into the body via the oral mucosa or the small intestinal mucosa or distributed to all relevant -destinations.

Our tip: Some people feel that the simultaneous use of coffee and Ginseng does no good to them and also the ancient Chinese avoid taking Ginseng with caffeinated drinks: They say that caffeine takes the energy from Ginseng. If possible, drink your morning coffee or black tea half an hour before or after taking your Ginseng.

Can I also take Ginseng more often or in higher doses?

People who are constantly exposed to increased stress or who suffer from severe chronic diseases, we recommend two 100-day cures per year or a constant Ginseng use. With a long-lasting Ginseng intake, you can reduce the dose to one capsule (or half a gram of Ginseng root) per day after a few months, depending on your personal feelings.

Before difficult exams or sporting challenges, you can increase the dose by two to three times for a few days.You increase the energy supply even more and allow the brain and muscles to perform at their best.

When should I start my Ginseng cure?

You can always start! If you want to protect yourself well against colds, we recommend starting in spring or autumn when the pathogens are all around. If you are just at the peak of your cold, you should not start with the Ginseng treatment; just wait a few more days to support your body in the recovery phase.

Ginseng against stress?

The phenomenon of stress is often cited as the reason for various diseases. Changes in the autonomic nervous system and in the hormonal balance, which occur during the stress reaction, can - at high intensity and long duration - certainly cause physical damage. This is proven, for example, for the development of cardiovascular diseases.

With the help of the Ginseng root, the body is able to react faster to the different stress triggers and to deal with them in a better way. The increased resistance delays exhaustion and stress-related diseases and possibly even prevents them. Ginseng causes less stress hormones to be formed and existing ones to be metabolized faster. In this context we also speak of the adaptogenic (adaptation) effect of Ginseng.

Ginseng for athletics?

Ginseng improves performance under stress: In our ancestors, physical top-performing was required when they suddenly faced an enemy and had to fight or when they had to escape. Today, the will to win, the shot from the starting pistol and the fans in the arena are the "stress factors". The performance of athletes increases with the Ginseng intake: Ginseng optimizes the metabolic processes, thus, active people can make better use of their energy. Specifically, improved muscle oxygen uptake and utilization, increased heartbeat volume, and a decrease of lactose concentration in the blood were observed.

A healthy and safe way to boost your physical performance: Doping is out - Ginseng is in.

Does Ginseng help my brain?

Clearly yes - ginseng stimulates the brain. With the help of an "electroencephalogram" (EEG) one can measure which brain cells work and how intensively they do that. Biochemical laboratory studies show that the cells have an increased activity with increasing ginseng dose.

People and animals always performed better in performance tests with ginseng than without. Experiments with the elderly have also shown that under the influence of ginseng learning, concentration and response skills are improved and intellectual capacity increases.

Can I use ginseng to strengthen the immune system?

Although Ginseng has no direct antibacterial or antiviral activity, it does have a protective effect on various pathogens. Ginseng increases the number of white blood cells, which are responsible for the detection and defense of pathogens. The production of messengers, which are responsible for the communication within the "defense team", is also increased by Ginseng. With the help of Ginseng the body is well prepared against stress factors, in this case pathogens!

Ginseng for diabetes?

Type 2 diabetes usually have a congenital hyposensitivity to the body's own insulin. This "insulin resistance" is aggravated by obesity and lack of exercise, so that type 2 diabetes ("adult onset diabetes") is the result. In the case of a diabetic diagnosis, therefore, your Doctor usually recommends that you first: "Move and reduce your weight!"

That's not so easy - Ginseng gives you the power and energy you need to put the important advice of your Doctor into action.

As has been shown in studies, the Ginseng agents also directly cause a lowering of the elevated blood sugar level. A high blood glucose level is an imbalance condition in the body, a disorder that is recognized and counteracted by Ginseng.

Diabetes can not be remedied with Ginseng on its own, but its use in some cases allows a reduction in the usual antidiabetics and increases the general condition affected by the disease – so you can also prevent other complications associated with type 2 diabetes!

Please take also notice of our advice for diabetics!

Ginseng for cancer?

The importance of Ginseng as a supplement to conventional cancer therapy and in prevention should not be underestimated. The general strengthening effect of Ginseng on the organism and on the resistance of the body, which has been known for more than 2000 years, is especially important in the treatment and prevention of cancer. Recent studies from Korea show that regular use of Ginseng can significantly reduce the risk of cancer. This effect is due to the mode of action of Ginseng: He reinforces the protection against external factors that can promote the development of cancer.

In cancer therapy Ginseng strengthens the weakened organs and the poor immune system. The side effects of radiation and chemotherapy are mitigated; blood formation in the bone marrow is promoted.

Ginseng for high blood pressure?

Generally speaking: Ginseng stabilizes the blood pressure in a very individual manner. It compensates aberrations upwards and downwards. Concerning blood pressure it shows again the "adaptogenic", regulating effect. Although research confirms this bi-directional effect of Ginseng, Chinese medicine literature also suggests that Ginseng is better avoided in high blood pressure patients, or only under medical supervision. Therefore, we also recommend: Inform your Doctor about the use of Ginseng, and let your blood pressure check regularly especially during Ginseng intake. Perhaps you may also be able to reduce the dose of one or the other drug due to the Ginseng intake.

Ginseng in times of post-menopausal complaints?

In the menopause, the body is affected by hormonal imbalances, which has a significant effect on the general well-being of many women. Many women report beneficial effects of Ginseng: Mood swings subside, hot flashes and feelings of weakness occur much less frequently or in a alleviated form. Unfortunately, there are no reliable scientific studies, but it is always worth a try, especially considering the many other health benefits of the ginseng root.

Ginseng for erectile dysfunctions?

Ginseng was for millennia and still is today considered an aphrodisiac: He should strengthen the potency of men and increase their fertility. In fact, ginseng helps with sexual problems: Ginseng makes you more resilient, relaxes, stimulates and tones your whole body via the hormone system ginseng influences sperm production in the testes. In healthy as well as in sick, the number of sperms and their mobility significantly increases.

CONSUMER INFORMATION USE

This book is just a guide on the health benefits of Ginseng. It is not a specific medical advice intended to replace information or advice from your medical personnel. It is only your healthcare provider that fully understands your health challenges and as such, has the knowledge and requisite training to provide the right and necessary medical advice for you.

In essence, you should not rely on the information provided by this guide to decide whether or not to use or accept your medical personnel's advice regarding the use of any natural products or similar treatments, therapies or life-style choices.

Please also note that this book does not recommend or endorse any natural products or similar treatments, therapies or life-style choices as safe, effective or approved for treating any health condition whatsoever.

Furthermore, this book does not encapsulates all information about natural products, possible uses, directions, warnings, precautions, interactions, advserse effects or riks applicable to you. You are advised to consult your medical personnel for complete information about your heath status and available or recommended treatment options.

About the Author

Dr. Alice Onofua is a Professor of bology at the University of California. She received her M.D in penn state and eventually earned her spot at Pennsylvania hospital in the emergency center. She has devoted much of her life to the study of human anatomy and physiology, and has pioneered early learning research through Anatomy Education Research Institute (AERI). Dr. Alice is also a publisher. Her articles on different subjects about how body system can grow naturally without the effect of using drugs or checking medical centers have appeared in leading professional publications and her work has been profiled in hundreds of other media reports.

Acknowledgments

My appreciation goes to God Almighty for the

opportunity and wisdom he gave me to complete this

book.

Profound thanks to those who contributed one way or the

other to the success of this book.

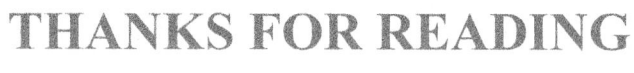

THANKS FOR READING